Sam's Secret Life

The Storybook Illustrated Guide to **OCD**

by Brian Wu

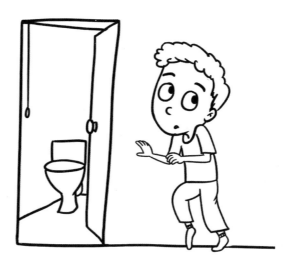

SiGuides
Mission and Meridian
South Pasadena, CA 91030
www.SIGuides.com

Disclaimers

This is a work of fiction. Names, characters, businesses, places, events and incidents are either the products of the author's imagination, or used in a fictitious manner. Any resemblance to actual persons, living or dead, or actual events is purely coincidental.

Although the author and publisher have made every effort to ensure that the information in this book was correct at press time, the author and publisher do not assume, and hereby disclaim any liability to any party for any loss, damage, or disruption caused by errors or omissions, whether such errors or omissions result from negligence, accident, or any other cause.

This book is not intended as a substitute for the medical advice of physicians. The reader should regularly consult a physician in matters relating to his/her health and particularly with respect to any symptoms that may require diagnosis or medical attention.

Storybook Illustrated Guides

Special Gift!

I'm glad that you took the time to read this, so I wanted to send you a special gift!

I want to give you free and useful resources on health (both for children and caregivers) and as list of tips for a happy, healthy life. Just add your email address to our list on SIGuides.com

You'll get immediately an email with our "Parent's Guide to Healthy Eating for Kids"!

If you have any comments, questions or want to give us some feedback, please write to brian@siguides.com

—Brian W. Wu

Founder of SIGuides

Storybook Illustrated Guides

www.SIGuides.com

Our Current Titles in English:

- The Day Jake Lost His Breath. The SIGuide to Asthma.
- Estelle's Winning Spirit. The SIGuide to Type 1 Diabetes.
- Joe Vs. The Ce-Monster. The SIGuide to Celiac Disease.
- The Zoo Flu Frenzy. The SIGuide to Influenza.
- Fort Applegate and the Battle of Wounded Knee. The SIGuide to Immune System
- Rufie's Amazing Journey. The SIGuide to the Cardiovascular System.
- Where Did my Bean Burger Go? The SIGuide to the Digestive System.
- Bobby's Bad Day. The SIGuide to ADHD.
- Sammi's New Normal. The SIGuide to Epilepsy.
- The World's Greatest Spy. The SIGuide to the Nervous System.
- Molly's Baby Brother. The SIGuide to Autism.
- Susie and the Great Big Giant Apple. The SIGuide to Weight Loss.
- Emily's Best Gift Ever! The SIGuide to New Babies.
- Don't Let the Bedbugs Bite! The SIGuide to Good Sleep.

Our Current Titles in Spanish:

- El día que Jake perdió su aliento. La historieta ilustrada que es una guía para el asma.
- El espíritu ganador de Estela. La historieta ilustrada que es una guía para la diabetes tipo 1.

Our Upcoming Titles:

- SIGuide to Type 2 Diabetes
- SIGuide to the Respiratory System
- SIGuide to the Renal System

Table of Contents

Tips for Coping with OCD

OCD can be difficult to manage, both for the parent and child. Here are some tips for coping with it on a day-to-day basis.

General Tips

Here are some general tips for parent and kids to cope with OCD.

• Keep in mind that OCD truly is a disorder; it cannot be helped by kids "trying to be better". It does require therapy and sometimes medication to help cope with the condition.

• OCD can be frustrating to live with as a parent. It sometimes helps to keep in mind that it is the OCD and not the child that is the source of the frustration!

• Family and emotional support can be extremely important for OCD kids.

• Try to lead as normal and structured a home life as possible; do not let the OCD become the "boss" of the home!

• Even with medication and therapy, improvement will come at different rates for different children. Try not to compare your child's progress with that of other children. Give praise for even small accomplishments, as this is great positive reinforcement for desired behavior.

Use This Book

Use this book as a means of getting your child interested in learning and as a teaching tool.

Chapter 1: Dude, Where's My Soap?

It was six-thirty in the morning in early January. It was that time of year that most kids dreaded. It was the first week back to school after the Christmas vacation that was spent opening presents, visiting Grandma and Grandpa's house, and eating way too many pieces of pie!

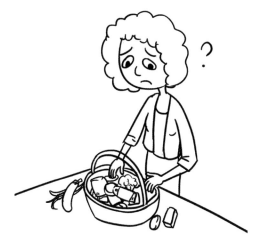

It was still dark outside, but Sam was already up, even though his little brother Pete was still fast asleep in the room across the hall.

Sam heard him snoring blissfully away as he himself padded down the hall to the bathroom. He knew that if he were to sneak into Pete's room right now, that Pete would be curled up in a ball under his Transformers blanket with his head resting against his Transformers pillow, and he would be drooling all over Optimus Prime.

Sam shook his head a little as he slipped quietly into the bathroom. Turning on the water in the sink just a little, so his mom couldn't hear it, he took a few big squirts out of the antibacterial soap dispenser and washed his hands thoroughly, under the nails, up his wrists and between his fingers. He knew how to wash hands.

He sighed a little after he rinsed his hands. Sam felt pretty anxious about things a lot, but slipping into the bathroom and giving his hands a good scrub-down to make sure they were nice and clean seemed to help him a lot.

He turned the taps off, careful to do it with a paper towel. After all, who knew what kind of germs would be on those knobs? Everybody in the house touched them. And Sam knew that there had been some workman in here the other day. They had come in to fix the ceiling fan in his parents' room. Sam just knew that they had come in here and washed their hands too!

Sam shuddered. The very thought seemed to give him a sick, wiggly, uncomfortable feeling right in the pit of his stomach!

He tried to brush those thoughts away. He had a lot of thoughts like that. Weird thoughts. Sometimes they were scary thoughts. It seemed to him that the only thing that made them better was to wash his hands a lot and make sure he kept away from all those nasty germs!

He opened the bathroom door a crack and looked both ways down the hall.

There was no one.

So, quick as a flash, Sam ran down the hall and back to his room again, closing the door behind him and diving into the bed. When his mom came in ten minutes later, he pretended to be asleep. She came in and shook him a little to wake him up.

Sam's mom, Lorraine, was a pretty woman. She had skin the color of a cup of coffee with cream in it, which Sam had inherited, and very dark curly hair which she usually wore in a big messy bun on top of her head.

Sam loved his mother very much. But he didn't want her to know that he snuck into the bathroom every morning. Sometimes he would do this several times at night, when he got home from school, and even *at* school if he had the chance, just to keep his hands clean. He didn't think she would like that, somehow, and he didn't want her to think he was a freak or something.

"Go ahead and get dressed. Breakfast will be ready in about ten minutes, okay?"

"Okay," said Sam, pretending to yawn and look sleepy.

She gave him a smile as she left the room. Sam, truly tired, dragged himself out of bed to get dressed.

The mornings were kind of rough on Sam. He felt like he had to get into the bathroom several times to make sure that his hands were truly clean and germ-free, but it was a busy household and even getting access to the bathroom could be kind of hard. He had given his hands a really good scrub down that morning!

Sam thought to himself, *"Did I really clean them well enough though? I mean, I think I did, but germs are everywhere! I have to make sure I really scrub down good. I don't want to get sick with some horrible disease and die!"*

He worried about this on his way down to breakfast, where his mother was rummaging around in the grocery bags from their shopping trip and his father was going through some of the bills for the month.

"Hmmm, that's weird," his mom said, rummaging deeply into one of the grocery bags, "You know, I could've sworn that I bought some more soap yesterday and another bottle of that hand sanitizer, too. I bet they forgot to put it in the bag or something. Oh, that's so irritating!"

"Do you want to know what's *really* irritating?" Sam's father asked. "This water bill. That's what's irritating. It seems like for the past few months, it just keeps going up and up! I might have to give our plumber a call. This is getting ridiculous. I wonder if there's a leak under the house?"

"Oh, dear, I hope not." Lorraine gave a sigh, then smiled at Sam and set down a hot plate of scrambled eggs, turkey bacon and whole-wheat toast. "There you are, sweetie."

Sam took the plate with a mumbled, "Thanks, mom", but he wouldn't look at her as he sat down to eat.

He knew where the soap and hand sanitizer had gone to. And he also knew why their water bills were getting so high, and it wasn't some leak in the basement!

Sam really loved his parents. He even loved Pete, when Pete wasn't being totally annoying, that is! He wanted to talk to them sometimes about how worried he was that he would get sick. He also worried that they would get sick! Even though his dad worked at the local hospital, they just didn't seem to realize how dangerous it was out there!

But something always held him back. He knew that other kids in his class, for instance, didn't worry about germs the way he did. They didn't care at all really! As a matter of fact, at lunch yesterday he'd seen some little first grader drop a tater tot on the floor and then pick it up and put it in his mouth off of the floor! Sam had nearly been sick to his stomach just thinking about it.

So, when his mom asked him if he was ready to drive to school, he gave a guilt little smile. "Be ready in a minute, mom. But first I..."

"...have to go to the bathroom?" his mother asked, smiling and shaking her head. "I swear, Sam, you have a more active bladder than any other child I know!"

Sam barely heard her, though. He raced up to the bathroom, grabbed the soap and turned on the water...

Chapter 2: When it All Began

A As they were driving to school, Sam was a bit thoughtful. He looked out the window and watched the familiar houses pass by on their way to Sunnybrooke Elementary. He was thinking about the day last fall when his life began to change, the day when Nurse Dumphrey had come to class to talk to them about the flu that was making its rounds through the entire school. Many students and teachers were out sick.

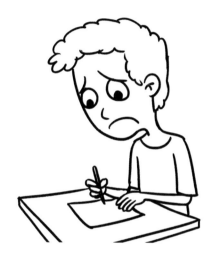

One of their classmates, Sarah, had actually been put in the hospital. When the other kids heard about this, they got pretty nervous. When Nurse Dumphery got up in the front of the class, Sam remembered that one of the girls, Susie, had raised her hand and asked the nurse if Sarah was going to die.

The class had gotten really quiet and Sam felt a sick, scared queasy feeling in the pit of his tummy.

He couldn't imagine dying when you were in third grade because of a nasty germ!

Sam hadn't even thought about that before and the idea really, really scared him.

Nurse Dumphrey shook her head. "I actually talked to Sarah's parents. She is doing a lot better and the doctors think she might even be able to come back to school tomorrow."

The class cheered.

"But," the nurse continued, looking serious, "Sarah did get really, really sick. Fortunately, very few of flu cases are that serious. To answer your question honestly, Susie, in some very rare cases, children can die from the flu."

The class got silent again.

"However," said the nurse brightly, "The great news is that there is a lot we can all do to stop from getting sick. Does anyone know what the best way to keep from getting the flu is?"

"Wear a mask?" Jimmy asked hesitantly.

"That's a very good guess, but the answer's much simpler than that. Does anyone else want to try? No?

Well, the best way to keep from getting sick, especially with the cold or the flu, is to wash your hands!"

Then she had showed them how to wash their hands properly so that they could be sure they were clean and also told them about hand sanitizer and how, though hand-washing was still the best, the sanitizer could protect them as well during the times when they could not wash.

Sam had always been the kind of kid who worried about things. But ever since Sarah had gotten sick and the nurse had said that they could actually *die* from the flu, he had been worried even more. And now he found himself thinking about it practically *all* the time.

Sam was still thinking about this as his mom dropped him off for school and he headed to class. He got there a few minutes before the bell rang. Sam was *always* early, so he could get into the restroom and give his hands a good scrub-down before class began. He also, if he had time, would wipe down his desk and pencils and things with some sanitizing wipes he had bought from the store with some of his allowance money.

Sam often spent his allowance money on stuff like that without his parents knowing about it. He felt bad that sometimes he couldn't go to the movies or stuff with his friends because he had already spent his allowance, but on the other hand, if it kept him safe, Sam figured it was worth it.

The bell rang. Jimmy, the boy who sat across the aisle from him came in, sat down and gave Sam a wave and a smile.

Sam waved back but didn't say anything. Sam got along pretty well with the other kids in the class. He didn't get teased or anything, but he didn't have any really close friends. For one thing, Sam didn't like to play basketball or baseball because he was worried about getting germs from the ball or bat... everyone had touched those! Sam knew that most of the other kids were *not* good about washing their hands, even after they went to the bathroom! Ew!

Sam also didn't like to go to other kids' houses or have a friend over for the same reason. If anyone came into his room, he got worried about germs they might be bringing in with them. If he went over to someone's house, he worried constantly if the place was clean or not, and usually had to wash his hands even more often than usual.

Jimmy was a pretty cool guy, though, so Sam did give him a smile as Mrs. Phelps came into the room.

"All right, class, are you ready?" she sang out. "It's time for our English test!"

Sam froze right there in his chair. He had been kind of distracted lately and didn't always pay attention when Mrs. Phelps read the book to them during English class.

The story she was reading was called, *The Lion, the Witch and the Wardrobe*, and Sam thought it was a pretty cool story so far, but he knew he didn't always listen the whole time she read.

"Okay, get out a piece of paper and label it from one to ten. This is going to be a short answer test, I just want to see what you've picked up from the reading. Are you ready?"

No! Sam thought to himself. He didn't say it out loud, though. He was sweaty and felt like his heart was beating too fast. He hated pop quizzes because they really stressed him out.

"Number one... what is the name of the youngest sister in this book?" Mrs. Phelps asked.

Lucy! Sam thought. He knew that one, at least! He wrote it down quickly.

"What is the name of the other land that Lucy discovers?" Mrs. Phelps asked next.

Nambia? Nu – Narn –? It was on the tip of Sam's tongue, but he just couldn't remember it. He started sweating a little more, and then one of those thoughts he got sometimes popped into his head before he could stop it.

Are my hands really clean? What if they're not? I might have brushed them on something and didn't even realize it! I don't want to get sick and die!

He knew Mrs. Phelps was pretty strict about not opening bags or getting up during the test in case someone tried to cheat. But he just couldn't help it as he reached down into his bag, took a few big squirts of the hand sanitizer, and rubbed it vigorously all over his hands. It stung a little. Sam's hands were always a little dry since he washed them so much, but Sam felt better right away. He gave a little sigh of relief and even finished the quiz without getting too many answers wrong.

When she came to collect his paper, though, Mrs. Phelps gave him a strange look. "Sam, I want you to stay for a few minutes when the bell rings for recess. I need to talk to you, ok?"

Sam nodded miserably. He was in trouble, he just knew it!

Chapter 3: Sam's Backpack Gives Him Away

"After Mrs. Phelps had picked up all the tests, she read them another chapter from the book, but although the story seemed to be getting really exciting, Sam barely paid attention.

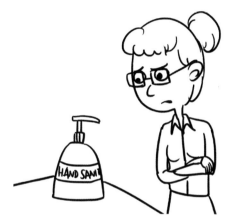

He didn't know what Mrs. Phelps wanted to talk to him about, but he knew it couldn't be good. Had she seen him getting into his bag during the test? He wasn't sure, but he knew like all teachers and moms, it seemed like she had eyes all over her head sometime and could see in about five directions at once.

He broke out into a sweat again. He really wished that the bell would ring for recess, so she could just yell at him and get it over with, if that was what she was planning to do. The waiting part was just rotten!

And for some reason, he kept worrying that his hands really weren't as clean as they should be, so when Mrs. Phelps seemed wrapped up in the story, he reached down into his bag and gave the hand sanitizer another squirt. He knew it wasn't as good as washing his hands, but it was a lot better than being totally unprotected!

Mrs. Phelps class had their recess after their first period, so when the bell rang, all the other kids filed out the side door to the playground, but

Sam stayed in his desk, waiting to see what Mrs. Phelps was going to do to him.

She came down the aisle, sat down in the desk in front of Sam, and turned around to face him. She didn't look mad or anything and Sam gave a little inward sigh of relief.

"Sam, I wanted to talk to you for a moment. I saw you rummaging around in your bag during the test and I wanted to talk, just you and me. I wanted to ask you, well, if you were cheating. Before you say anything, I want you to know that it will be much better if you just tell me about it now."

Sam looked up startled, "No, Mrs. Phelps, honest! I wasn't cheating, I swear!"

But he still felt really guilty. He *hadn't* been cheating, but there was that big bottle of hand sanitizer that he'd stolen out of his mom's grocery bag that he knew he shouldn't have, and some of that guilt must have shown on his face, because Mrs. Phelps said quietly.

"Well, would it be okay if I looked in your bag, Sam? I'd feel better if I knew you didn't have any notes or anything in there."

"Yeah, sure!" Sam practically shoved the bag at her. Hey, she was looking for notes or the book, not a bottle of sanitizer! He didn't think it would hurt anything for her to have a peek.

She looked in his bag for a moment then glanced quickly down at his hands before Sam could tuck them into his pockets. They were red and chapped and Sam had gotten pretty good at hiding them, but he got the feeling he wasn't fast enough to avoid her eagle eye. "I see."

Her expression had changed and Sam couldn't figure out what she was thinking from her tone of voice.

"Well, Sam, I don't see anything in here about the book so I don't think there was any problem about cheating. And I think it'd be a shame for you to miss all of recess, so why don't you go out and play, ok?"

"Okay." Sam heaved huge sigh of relief as he headed out the side door. He really liked Mrs. Phelps and he was glad that she didn't think he was a cheater. He didn't particularly like recess, either. He usually sat on the bench in the corner of the schoolyard and watched the other kids playing on the swing-set or monkey bars, but he knew that things like that were covered in germs, so matter how much fun they looked.

Sometimes, though, as he watched Jimmy and some of his friends swinging, he kind of wished he didn't worry about getting sick all the time. He wished he could just go over there and get on the swings with the rest of the kids and just be *normal*. But, he knew if he did that, he'd just start worrying about stuff all over again and wouldn't enjoy himself, anyway. So what was the point?

To his surprise, he found himself starting to cry, but he stopped himself and wiped his tears away with the back of his hand before anyone else saw them. It just wasn't a good day today, he thought, and that was all there was to it.

He was glad when the bell rang to go back in. He really hoped the rest of the day would go by fast and he could just get away and go home. He was just about to go back in when he looked up and saw the very last person he wanted to see walking towards him across the playground... Nurse Dumphrey!

She had already caught his eye so he couldn't pretend just to ignore her and walk away because he knew that it would be really rude. He looked down at his feet and didn't look up again when she stopped beside him.

"Sam?"

Sam nodded, still staring at the ground.

"Sam, I'd like you to come with me, okay?" Nurse Dumphrey had a nice, soft sort of voice. Just listening to it made Sam feel a little better at least. Even though he really didn't want to, he followed Nurse Dumphrey back inside the school.

He didn't know where they were going. But, he had a feeling he wouldn't like it when they got there.

Chapter 4: In Which Sam's Secret Life Isn't So Secret Anymore

As he followed Nurse Dumphrey from the playground into the school, Sam had that tight, queasy feeling he got sometimes in the pit of his stomach and he really, really wanted to pop into the restroom to give his hands a quick wash.

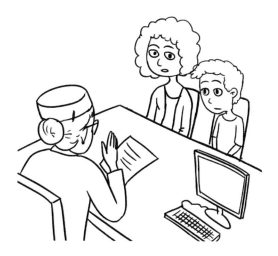

"Nurse, can I—?" he began.

She turned around to face him and her smile was kind, but firm. "I think you've washed your hands enough for right now, Sam." She glanced down at his red, chapped hands.

That was when Sam knew he was busted. Mrs. Phelps's eagle eyes had not missed the significance of the hand sanitizer. Geez, what was it with teachers and moms? They always saw all the things you wished they wouldn't!

Sam's stomach froze when he got to Nurse Dumphrey's office. His mom was there! Even worse, it looked like she had been crying.

Sam felt his stomach twist up into a knot of misery. He loved his mom a lot and he didn't like to see her worried or upset, which is exactly why he hadn't wanted to talk to her about all his weird, crazy thoughts in the first place!

It looked like his cover was blown sky-high! He sat down with a sigh, staring at the floor. He felt too embarrassed to look at his mom.

"Sam, your mom and I have been talking for a bit and, well, to be honest with you, we're worried about you. I know it can be kind of embarrassing to talk about things like this sometimes, but before we say anything else, we want you to know that you're not in trouble and that none of us are angry with you."

"That's exactly right, Sam." Sam's mom's voice still sounded like she had a cold or something, but she reached over and squeezed his shoulder, anyway. "Your dad and I both love you very much. You know that, don't you?"

Sam nodded, his face turning red and hot. He was still too embarrassed to look up.

"Your dad wanted to be here, too, but he's already on his flight for his business trip. He sends his love and he will be back on Friday," his mom went on.

Sam squirmed some more, "That's okay," he mumbled. That really was okay with Sam. He hated all this fuss and was glad that there weren't more than just two grown-ups to deal with!

"So, Sam, do you wash your hands a lot?" the nurse asked gently.

"Um, yeah," said Sam. He figured there was no point in trying to cover it up now. The cat was out of the bag as well as the hand sanitizer bottle!

"How often?"

"Um, I dunno." Sam thought about it for a moment, then went on. "Well, I wash as soon as I get up, and usually once or twice more before breakfast. As soon as I get to school, I wash them again. It's harder in class, you know, so I wash between classes or at recess, or I just use that," he gestured to the bottle of sanitizer that was sitting on the corner of the nurse's desk.

"Do you ever get up at night to do it?"

"Um, yeah. Sometimes I wake up at night for no reason and I'll go and do it then," Sam answered. He felt a slightly more relaxed now. Even if it was embarrassing, it felt good to get it off his chest!

"That's a lot of hand-washing, isn't it Sam?" The nurse asked softly.

"Yeah, I guess so." Honestly, up until that moment, Sam hadn't thought about just how much he really did wash up. When he wasn't washing, he thought about how much of his time he spent worrying if he'd washed enough. That really was kind of weird, now that he thought about it!

"Why do you wash your hands so much?"

"I dunno, just because." Sam muttered. He felt embarrassed again.

"Are you sure you don't know?" Nurse Dumphrey asked again.

"I, well…" Sam spluttered a bit, then burst out, "…I don't want to get sick and die!"

"Oh, Sam," he mother squeezed his shoulder again. Sam could tell she had started to cry again, but he had his eyes fixed on the nurse. "I started getting scared this past fall when the flu started going around and all those teachers and kids got sick. You came around and told us how Sarah had gone to the hospital and almost died. Then you said that washing our hands was the best way to keep from getting sick!"

The nurse sighed, "It is the best way, Sam. But, the fact that you're really worried about this and that you're washing your hands all the time is what makes your mom and I concerned."

"What do you think is wrong?" his mom asked.

"You'll have to go into Sam's doctor and talk about this to be sure. I suspect that, from what Sam is telling me, he has **Obsessive Compulsive Disorder**."

"What the heck is that?" asked Sam. He never thought there'd be a name for worrying and washing your hands a lot!

"It's a disorder where the person gets worrying or upsetting thoughts in their head that won't go away. These thoughts are called *obsessions*," the nurse explained.

25

Sam nodded. That was a good way of describing how ho felt about germs. He tried not to worry about them, but he just couldn't help it!

"Those obsessions lead to repetitive actions, in this case, your hand-washing, that the person feels they have to do to make their obsession go away."

Sam nodded again. He always felt less worried once he was done washing his hands.

"The biggest problem with this disorder is how much it can disrupt everyday life… school, having friends, getting enough sleep… anything can be affected by these obsessions and compulsions."

Sam's mother was very quiet for a moment. Then she said quietly, "Sam never asks to have anyone over to the house. He also never wants to go to anyone else's place, either. I always thought it was because he was shy, but…"

"…I just don't want to get sick," Sam finished for her. It was true.

"So, nurse, what can we do about this?" Sam's mom asked, "Is it something that his father and I did? Did we make a mistake?"

The nurse shook her head. "We really don't know why OCD happens. It can happen to kids if they have a family history of it, but it can also happen to kids who have no family history at all. As I said, you'll want to talk to the doctor about it. Sometimes doctors will prescribe medications to help control these thoughts and feelings, but sometimes therapy alone can work. Dr. Robertson works downtown and he has seen many kids with this issue. The therapy can really help."

"What will he do, exactly?" Sam asked nervously.

"Well, one type of therapy is called *exposure and response therapy*. This means that the therapist will expose Sam to things that he is worried about or afraid of. In this case, the fear is germs. The doctor will help him to build up a healthier, different response to this other than the compulsive hand-washing. It might take some time, but I know Dr. Ross has used it on other students from Sunnybrooke in the past and had good results."

"What do you think, Sam? Do you want find out if Dr. Ross can help us?"

Sam thought for a moment. He remembered how he felt earlier in the day, watching the kids playing on the swing-set. He really had wanted to go over and play, too, but he just worried about the germs too much! He liked the idea of being able to hang out with the other kids without those scary thoughts nagging him all the time.

"Yeah," he said after thinking about it for a few minutes. "Yeah, let's do it!"

Chapter 5: Six Months Later

It was the middle of the summer now. The days were longer and the weather was warm. Sunnybrooke Elementary was closed until the beginning of September, with a cheerful sign out front that said "See You in the Fall!" All the kids in town groaned or made faces at it whenever they walked by it!

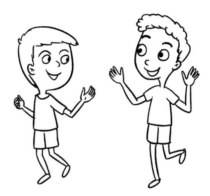

It had been a pretty good summer for Sam. He had been seeing Dr. Robertson for about six months now. He had started taking paroxetine, which the doctor said would help make him worry less, and he went in for sessions twice a week. The doctor felt that he was making good progress.

Sam felt that way, too. He was sleeping through the night, now that he wasn't jerking awake in the early hours of the morning worrying about washing his hands!

It wasn't that Sam didn't worry about germs at all anymore. He still did worry sometimes. When he got stressed about something, he worried even more. But Dr. Robertson was showing him ways he could deal with that worry instead of washing his hands twenty times a day! Sam's hands were actually getting back to normal now and it was the first time in months that they hadn't felt dry and chapped.

One of the things that Sam liked best about this summer was that he had a new friend. A few weeks ago, Sam had seen a moving van pull up in front of the house next door, a house that had been for sale since the end of the spring. A mover got out and began bringing boxes and pieces of furniture in, and it turned out to be Jimmy and his family!

Jimmy had given a big grin when he saw who his new neighbor was going to be. He had waved and come over to the fence which separated the two yards. Sam had come over, too.

"Wow, Jimmy! I didn't know you were moving!" Sam said, watching his with wide eyes.

Jimmy grinned, "My mom's going to have a baby, and guess what? About a month or so ago, the doctor told her she's going to have twins! She was pretty freaked out and started asking my dad about finding a bigger house, and they finally settled on this one." He gestured to the house behind him. "And here we are!"

"Cool! Do you like it?" Sam asked. He hoped that they would like it and they would stay.

"Well, I kind of miss our old place. It had a really neat tire swing in back in a big oak tree, but I like this place, too! I get my own room now, and my brother and I are pretty happy about that! There's a clubhouse in the back, too, and mom says it's all mine! My big brother Mike says he's too old for that, anyhow, and Mom thinks I'll need someplace to get away when the twins are born."

"Cool!" Sam said again, smiling.

"Hey, do you want to come over and see it?" Jimmy asked.

Sam hesitated for a moment. He didn't know if the house would be clean or not and…

He stopped himself. He knew that Dr. Robertson would be really proud of him if Sam went over to Jimmy's place. He could tell him all about it the next time they saw each other!

He thought to himself, "*Germs are not the boss of me! Germs are not the boss of me! Germs are…*"

It worked. "Yeah, that'd be awesome. Let me go tell my mom and I'll be right back."

That had been the beginning of it. Now Sam and Jimmy were at each other's house most days! Sam was still nervous about having Jimmy over or going over to Jimmy's house once they moved in, but after a while, he had gotten more used to it and now he actually enjoyed having such a close friend.

He still did not like playing baseball or basketball, since touching the equipment still made him a little uneasy, but he had found something he was really good at... swimming! Jimmy's house had a big swimming pool in back and the two of them would go swimming most days, with either one of their moms watching them.

Sam found out he loved to swim! The water in the pool was super clean and he felt really good when he was in it.

Jimmy's dad was super cool, too! When he saw that they were both enjoying the swimming so much, he set up lanes down the length of one side of the pool. He and Jimmy would race each other and they had even started talking about trying out for the swim team once they got back to school in the fall.

One morning they had gone for a swim and were pretty well tired out. They were sitting at the table by the side of the pool with a big umbrella over it for shade while Jimmy's mom laid out in the sun to get a tan. She had made them a plate of sandwiches and a big pitcher of lemonade before she had come outside, and the two of them gulped the food down happily. Jimmy was telling him at the Burnside Upper Elementary School, where he and Sam would be going in the fall, that they had an Olympic-sized pool to practice in!

Jimmy, who was really talkative, chattered on. Sam was only half listening, as he watched the cool blue water of the pool and the big puffy clouds moving across the summer sky above them. He had a good friend now and had found something that he really loved to do. It was probably the best summer he had ever had!

There wasn't much else to say. Sam took one last, long, messy slurp of his lemonade. Life was good.

Glossary of Terms

Compulsions: Compulsions are repetitive behaviors which people with OCD use to help temporarily decrease their anxiety levels. In this story, Sam's compulsion was hand-washing.

Exposure and Response Therapy: Therapy where the person suffering from OCD is exposed to what stresses them and then they learn alternative ways to cope with that stress.

Obsessions: Obsessions are persistent, stressful thoughts or ideas that can lead to compulsions in those with OCD.

Obsessive-Compulsive Disorder: Obsessive-compulsive disorder is a mental health disorder characterized by persistent, stressful thoughts or fears (obsessions) which translate into repetitive actions (compulsions).

Helpful Resources

- **Obsessive Compulsive Disorder (Mayo Clinic):** This is a great introduction to all basics of the disorder, including its definition, signs and symptoms, diagnosis, risk factors and treatment.

  www.mayoclinic.org/disease-conditions/ocd/basics/defintion/con-20027827

- **Obsessive-Compulsive Disorder (National Institute of Mental Health):** This is similar to the patient education at the Mayo Clinic but more in-depth and also has a great section on the newest trends and discoveries in OCD research.

  www.nimh.nih.gov/health/topics/obsessive-compulsive-disorder-ocd/index.shtml

- **Obsessive-Compulsive Disorder (Kid's Health):** This site has three different versions aimed respectively at adults, teens and children and talks about the disorder in a way that makes it easier for children especially to understand. It is an extremely well-written site.

  www.kidshealth.org/parents/emotions/behavior/OCD.html

About the Author

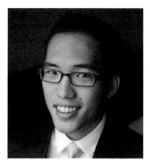

Brian Wu, a 7th year MD/PhD, is on track to finishing his PhD in 2014 and has a goal to becoming a Sports Medicine Physician with a focus on holistic care and treatment.

The idea for writing the Storybook Illustrated Guides first occurred to Brian as a fifth grader, when he wrote a story "Wacky Olympics and Body Wars", which is a personification of the immune system and how our bodies fight disease. Since then, the idea has matured over the years and the result is nothing short of astonishing. Brian has created a revolutionary series of books that raises the bar where children's health education is concerned. There's nothing else like the SIGuides on the market today.

Brian believes children should understand medical conditions they acquire, so that they can take good care of themselves and lead full lives. He has a way of writing about complex medical topics at a level that children comprehend. Brian understands the value of empowering children with diseases, enabling them to play an active role in their own treatment and recovery process.

Brian values the ability for all ages to learn from the power of stories. He has the passion to share his love of science and medicine through these stories with the world. The power of storytelling stems from the fact that stories can teach without overbearing. Learning comes naturally when engaging both logical and creative sides of the brain. The facts surrounding each disease appeal to the logical side, making the story engaging and the learning fun. Brian knows that if he can help even a single person then the project will be well worth it. Brian's interests include writing and entrepreneurship. He is married and loves his wife dearly.

Contact Brian Wu at brian@siguides.com.

More info on Brian can be found at http://www.brianwwu.com

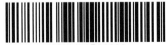
Printed in Great Britain
by Amazon.co.uk, Ltd.,
Marston Gate.